THE CANDIL FOR SENIORS

Defeating Candida Overgrowth in Seniors – A
Comprehensive Guide to Lifelong Wellness.

Linda Allen

TABLE OF CONTENTS

INTRODUCTION

How to Understand Candida Overgrowth

The goal of this chapter is to make the idea of Candida overgrowth clear to readers. A form of yeast called Candida is found naturally in our bodies, notably in the mouth, the digestive tract, and the skin. Candida normally coexists peacefully with other bacteria inside of us and doesn't create any problems. However, there are times when this equilibrium is upset, causing Candida to overgrow. Candidiasis is the medical term for this illness.

The following details are provided to readers in this chapter of the book:

Candida is defined as: It introduces Candida and describes it as a kind of yeast.

Candida's Function in the Body: When it's in the proper balance, candida benefits our systems, notably the digestive system and general wellness.

Symptoms of Candida Overgrowth: The warning signs and symptoms of excessive Candida growth are covered in this section. These signs may include troubles with the skin, the digestive system, and others.

Understanding Candida overgrowth is important because it enables people to identify when their Candida levels have gotten out of hand and need care. It lays the groundwork for understanding how to properly manage and treat this illness.

Reasons Seniors Are At Risk

This section of the book investigates why seniors—older adults—are more susceptible than younger people to developing Candida overgrowth. It explores a number of aging-related variables that may increase a senior's risk of developing this ailment. Among these elements are:

Decreased Immune System: People's immune systems tend to lose some of their ability to keep the body free from infections and imbalances as they age. Seniors may find it harder to control Candida as a result of their reduced immune systems.

Medications: Seniors often take many medicines, such as immune-suppressing drugs, steroids, and antibiotics, for a variety of medical issues. Some of these drugs have the potential to upset the body's microbiome, which might result in Candida overgrowth.

Dietary Practices: Candida overgrowth in older people may also be brought on by changes in dietary choices over time, such as an increase in the consumption of sugary or processed foods.

Chronic health conditions include the fact that seniors are more likely to suffer from chronic illnesses like diabetes or autoimmune diseases, which might foster the development of Candida.

CHAPTER ONE

CANDIDA EXPLAINED

What exactly is Candida?

Our bodies are home to a form of yeast called Candida. It is a tiny creature that lives on the skin, in the mouth, throat, stomach, and other areas of the body. Candida is often safe in tiny doses and even contributes to several healthy body processes.

But when the body's equilibrium with Candida is upset, issues might occur. This may result in a disease known as candidiasis, or the growth of the yeast Candida. Numerous health problems and symptoms may result from Candida overgrowth.

The body's natural microbiome, which includes a variety of bacteria, viruses, and fungi that exist both within and on the exterior of the body, includes Candida. These microbes contribute to maintaining health when they are in the proper balance. However, certain elements, such as a compromised immune system, the use of antibiotics, or a diet rich in sugar, may break this equilibrium, allowing Candida to grow and create health issues.

Candida overgrowth symptoms might include exhaustion, oral thrush (a fungal infection of the mouth), skin rashes, and stomach problems. In order to restore the equilibrium of the body's microbes, managing Candida overgrowth often entails dietary modifications, lifestyle modifications, and sometimes drugs. Recognizing when Candida becomes an issue and taking action to treat it requires knowledge about Candida and its function in the body.

Candida's Function in the Body

Yeast, namely Candida, is a kind that lives naturally in our systems and plays a number of crucial roles when everything is balanced out:

1. Digestion Help: Candida helps the body's digestive tract digest meals and assimilate nutrients. It facilitates the body's ability to digest carbohydrates and convert them into energy.

2. Keeping the Microbial Balance: In our gut, there are a variety of bacteria in addition to Candida. It coexists peacefully with other bacteria and fungi when everything is in balance. This equilibrium is necessary for intestinal health and general wellbeing.

3. Support for the Immune System: Our immune system and Candida interact. It aids in preparing the immune system to detect and react to future dangers, such as dangerous germs or fungi. Candida helps our body's defensive systems in this manner.

4. Vitamin Manufacturing: Certain Candida strains may create trace quantities of necessary vitamins, such as B vitamins. These vitamins are necessary for many biological processes, such as the creation of energy and the preservation of healthy neurons and skin.

But when Candida's delicate equilibrium is upset, issues might occur. An immune system that is weak, the use of antibiotics, or a diet that is high in sugar can all contribute to candida overgrowth, which may result in health issues. When Candida overgrows, it may produce symptoms and help with a variety of illnesses, including fungal infections, digestive issues, and more.

Maintaining the proper balance is thus essential to general health, even if Candida may play positive functions in the body when it's under control. When this equilibrium is upset, it might result in health issues that are linked to Candida and need attention

Symptoms of Candida overgrowth

A variety of symptoms may develop when the yeast Candida overgrows in the body. These signs might differ from person to person and could consist of:

1. Digestive Issues

- Constant gas and bloating
- Constipation or diarrhea
- Signs and symptoms similar to irritable bowel syndrome (IBS)
- Cramps or pain in the stomach

2. Symptoms in the mouth

- White, creamy spots appear on the tongue and in the mouth with oral thrush.
- Halitosis, or bad breath

3. Issues with the skin and nails

- Skin rashes that include peeling, itching, and redness
- Fungal skin, nail, or toenail infections (such as athlete's foot or nail fungus)
- Constant, irrational itching

4. Tiredness and weakness

- weakness in the muscles;
- generalized exhaustion;

- Feeling exhausted even after a good night of sleep

5. Repeated yeast infections

- Women's recurrent vaginal yeast infections
- Both men and women experience genital itching and pain.

6. Mood and mental health issues

- Mood swings
- Depression or anxiety
- Concentration issues or "brain fog"

7. Food Cravings for Sugar

- Prolonged and intense cravings for carbs and sweets
- A greater desire for sweet treats

8. Urinary Symptoms

- constant need to urinate
- Burning or pain while urinating

9. Allergic Reactions

- Allergies or sensitivities to different foods, chemicals, or environmental elements
- Hives or skin responses

10. Muscle and joint pain

- Joint stiffness and discomfort
- Muscle pain

It's important to keep in mind that other medical conditions, including Candida overgrowth, may also be the cause of these symptoms.

CHAPTER TWO

CANDIDA AND AGING

Considerations Related to Age

When we talk about the changes and difficulties that come with becoming older, we talk about age-related variables. These factors may all have an impact on a person's health, way of life, and overall happiness. The risk of developing Candida overgrowth increases with age due to a number of variables associated with becoming older. Some important aspects of old age include:

1. **Immunosuppression:** Aging often results in a weakening of the immune system. When the immune system is compromised, it becomes more difficult for the body to fight against infections and maintain a healthy microbial balance, which includes keeping Candida under control.

2. **Medications:** The need for careful drug management is heightened in the elderly population. Antibiotics and corticosteroids are only two examples of drugs that have the potential to upset the delicate equilibrium of the body's microbiome. Because of this upheaval, Candida overgrowth may be encouraged.

3. Alterations to the Diet: As people age, their tastes change, and they may start eating more processed and sugary meals. Such eating habits may foster a habitat favorable to the growth of Candida. The composition of gut bacteria is significantly influenced by one's diet.

4. Chronic Health Conditions: Chronic health conditions like diabetes, autoimmune diseases, or cardiovascular diseases are more likely to develop as people age. These conditions can alter the internal environment of the body, making it more conducive to Candida overgrowth.

5. Hormonal Changes: Hormonal changes are common in the aging process. For instance, hormonal changes brought on by menopause in women can have an impact on vaginal health and raise the risk of Candida-caused vaginal yeast infections.

It is important to have an understanding of these age-related characteristics since they explain why the elderly may be at a higher risk for Candida overgrowth and associated health problems. These considerations are important for elder healthcare because they allow for more individualized approaches to disease prevention and treatment.

Common Candida-Related Issues in Seniors

1. Oral Thrush: Seniors may develop oral thrush, a fungal infection characterized by white patches on the tongue, inner cheeks, and roof of the mouth. It can cause discomfort, difficulty swallowing, and altered taste perception.

2. Yeast infections of the vagina: Recurrent vaginal yeast infections may be more common in women, particularly postmenopausal older women. These infections may result in abnormal discharge, burning, and irritation.

3. Digestional Issues: Symptoms of digestive problems in seniors with Candida overgrowth include bloating, gas, abdominal discomfort, and changes in bowel habits (diarrhea or constipation).

4. Skin Infections: Seniors with Candida overgrowth may often have fungal skin infections, including ringworm, jock itch, and athlete's foot. These infections may result in pain, redness, and itching.

5. Chronic exhaustion: Seniors who have health problems associated with Candida often lament their ongoing exhaustion and lack of vitality.

6. Mental and Mood Health: Age-related changes in mood, anxiety, sadness, and difficulties focusing, or "brain fog," are all caused by candida overgrowth.

7. Muscle and joint pain: A Candida overgrowth may cause joint and muscular discomfort in certain elderly people.

8. Allergies and Sensitivity: Due to Candida overgrowth, seniors may become allergic or sensitive to certain foods, substances, or environmental factors.

9. Repeated urinary tract infections (UTIs): Seniors who have recurring UTIs may develop Candida, which may cause pain and frequent urination, among other urinary symptoms.

10. Dental difficulties: Candida-related difficulties may result in dental complications, such as tooth decay and gum infections.

11. Decreased Immune Activity: Seniors with candida overgrowth may have weakened immune systems, which makes them more susceptible to other infections and health issues.

12. Weight fluctuations: Some elderly people with Candida overgrowth may suffer changes in their weight, often having trouble shedding extra weight or experiencing unexpected weight reduction.

Not all seniors will encounter these problems, and the intensity of the symptoms might vary.

CHAPTER THREE

DIAGNOSIS AND TESTING

Identifying Candida Overgrowth

1. Recognize typical symptoms

- Start by becoming familiar with the typical signs and symptoms of Candida overgrowth, which might include:
- Digestive problems (gas, diarrhea, constipation, bloating)
- Oral thrush, which causes white mouth patches
- Eczema or fungus infections
- Weakness and exhaustion
- Depression, anxiety, or mood swings
- Recurrent yeast infections in the vagina (in women)
- Muscle and joint discomfort; recurrent sinus infections
- Concentration issues or "brain fog"

2. Self-Evaluation

Think about your own lifestyle and health. Consider the elements that may lead to Candida overgrowth, such as a high-sugar diet, regular use of antibiotics, or a compromised immune system brought on by aging or underlying medical issues. To keep track of any reoccurring or chronic symptoms, keep a symptom journal.

3. The Elimination Diet

Healthcare professionals could advise an elimination diet in various circumstances. This means avoiding suspected trigger items—such as sweets, processed foods, and alcohol—for a while to determine whether symptoms get better. If they do, it could indicate a problem with Candida.

Self-Assessment Tools

1. The Symptom Checklist: Make a note of the typical signs of Candida overgrowth, such as tiredness, mood swings, skin problems, and digestive difficulties. Make a note of the symptoms you encounter and their intensity to periodically evaluate your health. This might assist you in identifying any trends or changes over time.

2. Dietary Journal: Keep a journal of your eating patterns, noting the kinds of food you consume and how much sugar is in them. Keep track of which meals make your symptoms worse or trigger them. This may assist you in determining the likely dietary elements causing Candida overgrowth.

3. Questionnaires for Candida: You may measure your own risk of Candida overgrowth using a number of questionnaires connected to the condition that are accessible online or in books. The Dr. William Crook Candida Questionnaire is one that is often utilized. It queries about different symptoms and lifestyle elements.

4. Elimination Diet: Take into account using an elimination diet to see if it helps with your symptoms. This entails eliminating possible trigger items from your diet for a time (such as sugar and processed carbs) and then returning them gradually while keeping an eye on how your body responds.

5. pH evaluation: Measure the pH of your saliva and urine. Sometimes, Candida overgrowth may cause pH shifts. This approach should, however, be used in combination with other evaluation tools since it is not final.

6. Home Test Kits: There are several at-home test kits for finding Candida antibodies in your blood or stool. These tests may be able to shed some light on whether or not Candida is present, but as accuracy varies, findings should be treated with caution.

7. Watch for Recurrence: Pay attention to if your prior instances of Candida-related disorders (such as yeast infections) recurred regularly. Recurrences are often a sign of underlying Candida overgrowth.

CHAPTER FOUR

DIETARY GUIDELINES

What to Eat

It's critical to comprehend the rationale behind the Candida diet's selection of these items. Three things to think about are as follows:

- **Low-sugar**

Sugar is essential for Candida albicans' growth, colonization of your gut, and the development of the biofilms that shield it from your immune system (1). It makes no difference if the sugars you consume are natural (like in bananas) or artificial (like in candy bars). Only foods with a low sugar content are included in this list.

- **Gluten-free**

There is growing evidence that eating gluten-containing foods may harm one's health, even if they are not celiac (2). The gluten included in cereal, pasta, and bread may damage the connection between the cells lining your intestinal wall and result in persistent inflammation in your gut. Only grains and fake grains that are gluten-free are included on our list of Candida diet foods.

- **Anti-inflammatory**

One of the fundamental components of the Candida diet is avoiding inflammation. Because of this, we advise you to consume fewer processed meals, less coffee, and more fermented foods that have anti-inflammatory properties.

Candida-friendly foods

VEGETABLES WITHOUT CARBS

- Artichokes
- Asparagus
- Broccoli
- Brussels sprouts
- Cabbage
- Cauliflower
- Celery
- Cucumber
- Eggplant
- Garlic (raw)
- Kale
- Onions
- Rutabaga
- Spinach

- Tomatoes
- Zucchini

FRUITS WITH LOW SUGAR

- Avocado
- Lemon
- Lime
- Olives

GRAINS WITHOUT GLUTEN

- Buckwheat
- Millet
- Oat bran
- Quinoa
- Teff

HEALTHY PROTEINS

- Anchovies
- Chicken
- Eggs
- Herring
- Salmon (wild)
- Sardines
- Turkey

SOME DAIRY PRODUCTS

- Butter
- Ghee
- Kefir
- Yogurt (probiotic)

LOW-MOLD NUTS & SEEDS

- Almonds
- Coconut
- Flaxseed
- Hazelnuts
- Sunflower seeds

HERBS, SPICES, & CONDIMENTS

- Apple cider vinegar
- Basil
- Black pepper
- Cinnamon
- Cloves
- Coconut aminos
- Dill
- Garlic
- Ginger
- Oregano

- Paprika
- Rosemary
- Salt
- Thyme
- Turmeric

HEALTHY FATS & OILS

- Coconut oil (virgin)
- Flax oil
- Olive oil
- Sesame oil

NO-SUGAR SWEETENERS

- Erythritol
- Stevia
- Xylitol

FERMENTED FOODS

- Kefir
- Olives
- Sauerkraut
- Yogurt

DRINKS

- Chicory coffee

- Filtered water
- Herbal teas

Foods to Avoid

It's critical to comprehend the precise rationale for the inclusion of some items in the diet and the exclusion of others as you work to enhance the health of your gut. You may use the same reasoning to assess whether or not you can consume an item on your Candida diet if you come across one that isn't on the list.

For one of the three reasons listed below, every item on this list has been eliminated from the diet.

- **Foods with a lot of sugar**

Why does sugar matter so much to Candida albicans? In actuality, Candida needs sugar in order to develop, broaden its colonies, and create the protective biofilms that allow it to evade your immune system. In fact, 32% of the glucose in such biofilms is glucose (1). It doesn't matter whether this sugar comes from fruits' natural sugars or manufactured meals. Sugary snacks and fruits with a lot of sugar are thus not allowed.

- **Gluten-containing foods**

Not only those with celiac disease need to stay away from gluten. Going gluten-free was often considered a fad, but current research demonstrates that many individuals may improve their health by doing so (2). Gluten increases intestinal permeability, aggravates gut inflammation, and exacerbates Candida symptoms. Grain products containing gluten are therefore prohibited from the diet.

- **Foods that cause inflammation in the intestines**

There are other foods than gluten that might inflame the stomach. An excellent example would be refined vegetable oils. When not counterbalanced by meals high in omega-3 fatty acids, their high amounts of pro-inflammatory omega-6 fatty acids may lead to an increase in inflammation (3). Other items that might irritate and inflame the stomach lining include alcohol and coffee.

List OF Foods To Avoid

SUGARS AND SUGAR ALTERNATIVES

- Agave
- Aspartame
- Brown sugar
- Grain syrup

- Maple honey syrup
- Methanol Sugar

GLUTENOUS GREEN TEARS

- Barley
- Rye
- Spelt
- Wheat

SUGAR-RICH FRUITS

- Bananas
- Dates
- Fruit juices
- Grapes
- Mango
- Raisins

TOXIC FISH AND PROCESSED MEATS

- Processed meats
- Shellfish
- Swordfish
- Tuna

SOME DAIRY PRODUCTS

- Cheese

- Milk
- Cream

NUTS AND SEEDS WITH MOLD

- Nut butters made from rotten nuts

CONDIMENTS

- Barbecue sauce
- Horseradish
- Ketchup
- Mayonnaise
- Soy sauce
- White vinegar

PROCESSED/REFINED FATS & AND OILS

- Canola oil
- Fake 'butter' spreads
- Margarine
- Soybean oil
- Sunflower oil

ALCOHOLIC OR SUGARY DRINKS

- Beer
- Cider
- Liquors

- Spirits
- Wine
- Diet and regular soda
- Fruit juices
- Energy drinks

DRINKS WITH CAFFEINE (OPTIONAL)

- White tea Coffee

Balancing Nutritional Needs for Seniors

Making intelligent decisions to satisfy your body's changing nutritional demands as you age entails balancing your nutritional needs. The following recommendations can help you achieve dietary balance:

1. Prioritize a Diverse Diet:

Choose a variety of meals to ensure you obtain a wide range of nutrients. Your meals should include fruits, vegetables, whole grains, lean proteins, and healthy fats.

2. Place a Focus on Nutrient-Dense Foods:

Select meals that are high in nutrients yet low in calories. Give high-nutrient foods a higher priority, such as fruits, vegetables, lean meats, whole grains, and low-fat dairy products or dairy substitutes.

3. Watch the portion sizes:

Be mindful of portion quantities to prevent overeating. Because your metabolism may slow down as you get older, portion control is crucial for maintaining a healthy weight.

4. Protein Consumption:

Consume enough protein in your diet to promote general health and the maintenance of muscle mass. Lean meats, poultry, fish, beans, lentils, tofu, and low-fat dairy products are all excellent sources of protein for seniors.

5. Foods High in Fiber:

To promote digestive health and control cholesterol levels, include fiber-rich foods like whole grains, legumes, fruits, and vegetables in your diet.

6. Hydration:

Drink plenty of water. Seniors are more likely to experience dehydration, which may result in a number of health problems. Consume hydrating meals, including soups, fruits, and vegetables, as well as plenty of water.

7. Vitamin D and calcium:

Consume adequate calcium and vitamin D to promote the health of your bones. Leafy greens, fortified non-dairy milk, dairy products, and fish in cans with bones are all excellent sources.

8. Omega-3 Fatty Acids:

Include omega-3 fatty acid sources in your diet to maintain the health of your heart and brain. Walnuts, flaxseeds, chia seeds, and fatty fish (salmon, mackerel) are all great choices.

9. Reduce added sugars and sodium intake:

Limit your consumption of meals and drinks that are heavy in salt and added sugars. Heart disease and excessive blood pressure are only two conditions that may make it worse.

10. Special dietary considerations include:

Consult a dietician to develop a meal plan that suits your requirements if you have any dietary limitations or health issues (such as diabetes or food allergies).

11. Regular Meals:

Aim for consistent, well-balanced meals. Nutrient shortages and unstable blood sugar levels may result from skipping meals or depending only on harmful snacks..

CHAPTER FIVE

THE CANDIDA CLEANSE

Cleansing Protocols

The goal of cleansing procedures, often known as "detox" or "cleanse" regimens, is to remove toxins from the body, improve general health, and maybe treat particular health issues. The following are some crucial considerations regarding cleaning protocols:

1. Cleansing Methods: There are many different kinds of cleansing procedures, from quick juice cleanses to longer-term nutritional changes. Popular cleanses include:

- **Juice detoxes:** These include sticking to exclusively fresh fruit and vegetable juices for a certain amount of time.
- **Water fasting** is the practice of abstaining from all food and liquids for a certain period of time.
- **Elimination Diets:** Temporarily cutting out certain foods or dietary categories, such as sugar, dairy, or gluten, in order to discover any possible sensitivities or allergies.

- **Colon Cleanses:** Methods or supplements used to clear the colon of waste and toxins.
- **Whole Food Cleanses:** These include focusing on whole, unprocessed foods and avoiding processed foods, sugar, and caffeine.

2. Potential Benefits: Supporters of cleaning regimens claim that these might include better digestion, more energy, cleaner skin, and weight reduction. Cleanses may help eliminate toxins and reset the body, according to some supporters.

3. Scientific data: There is a lack of and sometimes conflicting scientific data to support the efficacy of cleaning treatments. While transitory gains may result from short-term dietary adjustments, there is no evidence to back up the long-term advantages of radical cleanses. Furthermore, the liver and kidneys of the body automatically detoxify the body, so most individuals may not need to undergo rigorous cleanses.

4. Side effects and Risks: Risks may be associated with extreme cleaning regimens, particularly those that include fasting or limiting one's nutrition. Nutrient shortages, muscle loss, electrolyte imbalances, and a poor effect on metabolism may be among these dangers.

Before beginning any cleaning program, it's important to speak with a healthcare professional, particularly if you have underlying medical issues.

5. Individualized Approach: There isn't a cleaning strategy that works for everyone. Each individual has a different ideal method for detoxing and maintaining health. What is appropriate for one person could not be for another. It's critical to take a customized strategy that takes into account your own health requirements, dietary choices, and medical background.

6. Hydroponics: During any cleansing, staying hydrated is essential. Water aids in the body's natural detoxification processes and aids in toxin removal.

Detoxification Methods

Detoxification techniques are strategies or routines designed to assist the body's inherent mechanisms for getting rid of waste and toxins. Here are a few typical detoxification techniques:

Hydration: One of the easiest and most efficient strategies to help detoxify is by drinking enough water. Water aids in the removal of toxins from the body via perspiration and urine. Aim to consume a lot of filtered, clean water throughout the day.

Healthy Eating: Consuming a nutrient-rich, well-balanced diet is crucial for promoting detoxification. Put an emphasis on complete foods, such as fresh produce, lean protein, whole grains, and healthy fats. Reduce your intake of processed meals, sugar, and synthetic chemicals.

Foods rich in fiber: foods rich in fiber, such as fruits, vegetables, and whole grains, may assist in digestion and encourage regular bowel movements, helping the body get rid of toxins and waste.

Support for the Liver: The liver is an important detoxifying organ. Broccoli, cauliflower, leafy greens, and beets are examples of foods that may improve liver function. Additionally, herbs that are known to promote liver function include milk thistle and dandelion root.

Exercise: Getting moving improves circulation and encourages sweating, which may help the body remove toxins. Additionally, regular exercise promotes general health and wellbeing.

Saunas and steam baths: Sweating is a natural method for the body to get rid of impurities. Saunas and steam baths may make you sweat. However, before using a sauna, those with certain medical issues or medicines should speak with a doctor.

Breathing activities: Deep breathing activities, such as diaphragmatic breathing or yoga, may encourage the evacuation of waste products from the body via the breath and help oxygenate the body.

Intermittent fasting: Some people use this type of fasting, which entails cycles of eating and not eating. This strategy could assist the body in reaching an autophagic state, where it recycles damaged cells and eliminates toxins.

Detox Diets: Some people engage in short-term detox diets that call for temporarily cutting out certain items like sugar or processed meals. Instead of being utilized as a long-term plan, these diets are often employed to detect food sensitivities.

Enemas or other colon cleaning techniques are sometimes used to flush toxins and waste from the colon. These should only be carried out under a healthcare professional's supervision.

Probiotics: Foods or supplements containing helpful bacteria known as probiotics may help maintain gut health, which is important for the body's detoxification processes.

Limit your consumption of alcohol and caffeine to help your liver and general health. Limiting these substances may help you feel better overall.

Reduction of Stress: Detoxification procedures might be impacted by chronic stress. Yoga and other stress-reduction practices, such as mindfulness meditation, may be beneficial.

The liver, kidneys, lungs, and skin are the body's primary natural detoxification organs, which should not be overlooked. Extreme detoxification regimens or fasts may not be safe for everyone and contain potential dangers. Before making any big dietary or lifestyle changes, always check with your doctor, particularly if you have underlying medical issues. The most efficient and long-lasting approaches to promoting your body's natural detoxification processes are often a balanced, whole-food diet and a healthy lifestyle.

Duration and Monitoring

Duration and monitoring are important considerations when engaging in detoxification methods or dietary changes. The duration of a detox program and the need for ongoing monitoring depend on the specific approach and individual goals. Here's what you should know:

1. Duration of Detox Programs:

- **Short-Term Detox:** Many detox programs are designed to be short-term, lasting anywhere from a few days to a few weeks. These short-term detoxes are often used to kickstart healthier habits, identify food sensitivities, or provide a reset for the body.

- **Long-Term Lifestyle Changes:** Detoxification doesn't necessarily need to be a short-term program. Long-term lifestyle changes that promote overall health and wellness can include ongoing practices such as eating a balanced diet, staying hydrated, exercising regularly, and managing stress. These are sustainable habits that support the body's natural detoxification processes over time.

2. Monitoring During Detox:

- **Self-Monitoring:** During a detox program, individuals should monitor how they feel physically and emotionally. Pay attention to changes in energy levels, digestion, mood, and any unusual symptoms. Keeping a journal of your experiences can be helpful.

- **Progress Assessments:** Regular assessments of your progress are important. If your goal is weight loss or specific health improvements, track relevant metrics such as weight, body measurements, or lab test results, if applicable.

3. Post-Detox Maintenance:

- **Transition to a Sustainable Diet:**** After completing a detox program, it's important to transition to a balanced and sustainable diet. Avoid returning to unhealthy eating habits or excessive indulgence in processed foods.

- **Lifestyle Integration:** Incorporate the positive habits you've developed during the detox into your long-term lifestyle. Continue to eat a nutrient-dense diet, stay hydrated, exercise, and manage stress.

- Periodic Detox Maintenance: Some individuals incorporate periodic, shorter detoxes (e.g., a weekend juice cleanse) into their routine as a way to maintain a healthy lifestyle. However, these should be approached with caution and tailored to individual needs.

4. Individualized Approach:

Detoxification needs and goals vary from person to person. What works for one individual may not be suitable for another. It's important to tailor your approach to your specific needs, preferences, and health conditions.

In summary, the duration and monitoring of detoxification methods depend on the specific approach and individual circumstances. Short-term detox programs can provide a reset and identify potential sensitivities, but long-term lifestyle changes that support the body's natural detoxification processes are often more sustainable and beneficial for overall health. Regardless of the approach you choose, consider seeking guidance from a healthcare provider or dietitian to ensure that it aligns with your health goals and is safe for you.

CHAPTER SIX

SUPPLEMENTS AND NATURAL REMEDIES

Probiotics and Prebiotics

Prebiotics and probiotics are two related substances that are essential for maintaining a balanced gut flora. An explanation of each follow:

Probiotics:

Live microorganisms known as probiotics—also referred to as "friendly" or "good" bacteria—offer a number of health advantages when taken in sufficient quantities. The microorganisms that live in your digestive system naturally are comparable to these helpful bacteria. Certain meals, dietary supplements, and fermented goods all contain probiotics.

Important facts regarding probiotics:

1. Health Advantages: Probiotics have been linked to a number of health advantages, including boosting immune function, enhancing digestive health, and even lowering the chance of developing certain gastrointestinal conditions.

2. Sources: Yogurt, kefir, sauerkraut, kimchi, miso, tempeh, and several varieties of pickles are common foods that contain probiotics. There are other probiotic supplements on the market.

3. Varieties of Strains: There are several strains of probiotics, and different strains may give different health advantages. Probiotic strains like Lactobacillus and Bifidobacterium species are two popular types.

4. Gut health: Probiotics may aid in preserving the gut's healthy balance of helpful microbes. For appropriate digestion and nutritional absorption, this equilibrium is crucial.

5. Probiotic dietary supplements: There are several different types of these supplements, including capsules, powders, and liquid versions. They are often used to increase probiotic consumption, particularly for those with certain health issues.

Prebiotics:

Prebiotics are dietary fibers and chemicals that are not digested and function as food for probiotics and other good bacteria in the stomach. Prebiotics are the compounds that feed and promote the development and activity of the live bacteria in the gut, while probiotics are the living bacteria themselves.

Important information regarding prebiotics:

1. Nourishing the Gut: Prebiotics work as a source of nourishment for the good bacteria in the stomach, which is the first benefit. They support the growth and efficient operation of these microorganisms.

2. Natural Resources: Prebiotics are included in many diets high in fiber. Garlic, onions, leeks, asparagus, bananas, oats, and chicory root are examples of common sources.

3. Digestive Wellness: Prebiotics may aid in the development of good gut flora and increase the creation of short-chain fatty acids, which offer a number of health advantages.

4. Synbiotics: Some products combine both probiotics and prebiotics and are known as synbiotics. These products aim to provide a comprehensive approach to gut health by delivering both beneficial bacteria and the nutrients they need to thrive.

5. Maintaining a balanced microbiota: Prebiotics are important for preserving a healthy gut microbiota, which is linked to general health and well-being.

Antifungal Herbs and Supplements

Antifungal herbs and supplements are natural substances that have properties capable of inhibiting the growth or spread of fungi, including Candida and other fungal infections. These herbs and supplements may be used to complement conventional treatments or as a preventive measure. Here are some commonly used antifungal herbs and supplements:

1. Garlic (Allium sativum): Garlic contains allicin, a compound known for its antimicrobial properties. It can help combat fungal infections when consumed in dietary form or as supplements.

2. Oil of Oregano (Origanum vulgare): Oil of oregano contains compounds like carvacrol and thymol, which have antifungal properties. It's available in both liquid and capsule forms.

3. Caprylic Acid: This fatty acid, often derived from coconut oil, is known for its antifungal properties. It can be found in supplement form.

4. Grapefruit Seed Extract: Grapefruit seed extract contains compounds that have demonstrated antifungal activity. It can be taken in liquid or capsule form.

5. Pau d'Arco (Tabebuia impetiginosa): Pau d'arco is an herb known for its antifungal properties, primarily due to compounds like lapachol. It can be consumed as a tea or in supplement form.

6. Black Walnut (Juglans nigra): Black walnut hulls contain juglone, a compound with antifungal properties. It's available as a tincture or in capsule form.

7. Berberine: Berberine is a compound found in various plants, including goldenseal and Oregon grape root. It has broad-spectrum antimicrobial properties, including antifungal effects.

8. Probiotics: While not directly antifungal, probiotics help maintain a healthy balance of gut bacteria, which can prevent fungal overgrowth in the digestive tract. Look for probiotic supplements with strains like Lactobacillus acidophilus and Bifidobacterium bifidum.

9. Coconut Oil: Coconut oil contains lauric acid, which has antifungal properties. It can be consumed in cooking or applied topically to affected areas

10. Aged Garlic Extract: Aged garlic extract is a specific form of garlic that may have enhanced health benefits, including antifungal properties. It's available in supplement form.

11. Neem (Azadirachta indica): Neem is an herb with natural antifungal and antibacterial properties. It's available in various forms, including capsules, creams, and oils.

12. Tea Tree Oil (Melaleuca alternifolia): Tea tree oil is often used topically for its antifungal properties. It should be diluted before application to the skin.

13. Echinacea (Echinacea spp.): Echinacea is known for its immune-boosting properties and may indirectly help the body fight fungal infections by supporting the immune system.

Nutritional Support

Support from nutrition is essential for preserving general health and wellbeing. It entails giving the body the vital nutrients it needs to sustain different physiological functions and perform at its best. Following are some crucial components of nutritional support:

1. Balanced diet: The cornerstone of nutritional assistance is a balanced diet. To guarantee that the body obtains a broad range of vital elements, including carbs, proteins, fats, vitamins, and minerals, it comprises a variety of meals from all dietary categories.

2. Macronutrients: These are the nutrients that must be consumed in large amounts and include lipids, proteins, and carbs. They give out energy and are necessary for all biological processes, including development and repair

3. Micronutrients: Although required in lower quantities, micronutrients such as vitamins and minerals are nonetheless crucial to good health. They participate in a number of physiological functions, such as metabolism, immunological response, and bone health.

4. Hydration: Proper hydration is vital for maintaining bodily functions. Water is necessary for digestion, circulation, temperature regulation, and the transport of nutrients and waste products.

5. Individualized Nutrition: Everybody has different nutritional demands depending on their age, gender, degree of exercise, and underlying health issues. It's crucial to have a specialized nutrition plan that is tailored to each person's unique requirements.

6. Nutritional supplements: Depending on their needs or certain health issues, people may sometimes need to take nutritional supplements. Vitamins, minerals, omega-3 fatty acids, and probiotics are typical supplements. A healthcare professional should be consulted before beginning any supplements.

7. Particular Dietary Considerations: Due to allergies, food sensitivities, religious convictions, or medical illnesses like diabetes or celiac disease, certain people may have particular dietary demands or limits. A diet that takes these factors into account is a component of nutritional assistance.

8. Meal Timing: The timing of meals and snacks may have an impact on blood sugar control and energy levels. Regular, well-balanced meals may help keep energy levels steady and help you avoid overeating.

9. Weight control: Whether it's weight reduction, weight maintenance, or muscle building, nutritional assistance is important for weight control. It's critical to strike a balance between calorie consumption and exercise.

10. Disease Prevention and Management: Healthy eating may aid in preventing and managing a number of chronic conditions, including heart disease, diabetes, and hypertension. Some diets, such as the DASH diet and the Mediterranean diet, were created expressly for the treatment and prevention of illness.

11. Mindful Eating: Practicing mindful eating entails being aware of your dietary preferences, hunger signals, and eating routines. It may discourage overeating and encourage a better connection with food.

One of the most important components of health and well-being is nutritional assistance. People may improve their physical and mental health, boost their immune systems, and lower their chance of developing chronic illnesses by giving their bodies the proper nutrients in the right proportions. Receiving individualized advice and suggestions based on your particular dietary requirements.

CHAPTER SEVEN

LIFESTYLE AND STRESS MANAGEMENT

Stress Reduction Techniques

Stress reduction techniques are strategies and practices that help individuals manage and alleviate stress, which is a common response to life's challenges and demands. Chronic stress can have negative effects on both physical and mental health, so it's important to incorporate stress-reduction techniques into your daily life. Here are some effective techniques:

1. Deep breathing: Deep, slow breaths can help calm the nervous system. Practice deep breathing exercises to reduce stress and anxiety.

2. Mindfulness Meditation: Mindfulness meditation involves focusing on the present moment without judgment. Regular practice can improve emotional well-being and reduce stress.

3. Progressive Muscle Relaxation: This technique involves tensing and then releasing different muscle groups in the body to promote relaxation.

4. Yoga: Yoga combines physical postures, breath control, and meditation to reduce stress, improve flexibility, and enhance mental clarity.

5. Exercise: Regular physical activity can release endorphins, which are natural mood lifters. Exercise also helps reduce stress hormones like cortisol.

6. Adequate Sleep: Prioritize getting enough sleep, as it plays a crucial role in managing stress. Lack of sleep can exacerbate stress levels.

7. Healthy Diet: A balanced diet with plenty of fruits, vegetables, and whole grains can support both physical and mental health, helping to manage stress.

8. Time Management: Effective time management and setting realistic goals can reduce stress related to work or daily responsibilities.

9. Social Support: Sharing your thoughts and feelings with friends or family can provide emotional support during stressful times.

10. Hobbies and Relaxation Activities: Engaging in hobbies and activities you enjoy can be a great way to relieve stress and take your mind off worries.

Sleep Hygiene

Sleep hygiene refers to a set of practices and habits that promote quality and restful sleep. Good sleep hygiene is essential for getting a good night's sleep, feeling refreshed, and maintaining overall health. Here are some sleep hygiene tips:

1. Consistent Sleep Schedule: Go to bed and wake up at the same time every day, even on weekends. This helps regulate your body's internal clock.

2. Create a Relaxing Bedtime Routine: Engage in calming activities before bed, such as reading, gentle stretching, or taking a warm bath.

3. Comfortable Sleep Environment: Make sure your sleep environment is comfortable and conducive to sleep. This includes a comfortable mattress, an appropriate room temperature, and minimal noise and light.

4. Limit Screen Time: Reduce exposure to screens (phones, tablets, and TVs) at least an hour before bedtime, as the blue light emitted can disrupt sleep.

5. Watch Your Diet: Avoid large meals, caffeine, and alcohol close to bedtime. These can interfere with sleep.

6. Physical Activity: Regular exercise can improve sleep, but avoid vigorous exercise close to bedtime.

7. Manage Stress: Use stress reduction techniques to manage anxiety and worries that can interfere with sleep.

8. Limit Naps: If you need to nap, keep it short (20–30 minutes) and earlier in the day.

9. Limit Exposure to Light: Exposure to natural light during the day and darkness at night helps regulate your body's sleep-wake cycle.

Both stress reduction techniques and good sleep hygiene practices contribute to improved overall health and well-being. By incorporating these habits into your daily life, you can better manage stress, enhance your sleep quality, and enjoy the benefits of a well-rested mind and body.

Exercise and Candida

While exercise is generally beneficial for overall health, it's essential to keep in mind that specific exercises do not directly target or treat Candida overgrowth. However, maintaining regular physical activity can help support your immune system, improve circulation, and promote overall well-being, which can indirectly contribute to better health and potentially aid in managing Candida overgrowth.

1. Walking

2. Jogging

3. Running

4. Cycling

5. Swimming

6. Hiking

7. Dancing

8. Aerobics

9. Yoga

10. Pilates

11. Tai Chi

12. Qigong

13. High-Intensity Interval Training (HIIT)

14. Jumping Rope

15. Stair Climbing

16. Rowing

17. Resistance Training

18. Bodyweight Exercises (e.g., push-ups, squats, lunges)

19. Weightlifting

20. Kettlebell Training

21. TRX Suspension Training

22. Barre Workouts

23. Water Aerobics

24. CrossFit

25. Zumba

26. Kickboxing

27. Indoor Climbing

28. Group Fitness Classes

29. Inline Skating

30. Parkour

Remember that the key to exercise's potential benefits for Candida overgrowth is consistency. Regular physical activity can help maintain a healthy body and immune system, which may indirectly support your body's ability to manage Candida. However, it should be used in conjunction with other treatments and lifestyle modifications if you are dealing with a Candida-related health concern. Always consult with a healthcare provider for a comprehensive treatment plan tailored to your specific needs.

CHAPTER EIGHT

RECIPES AND MEAL PLANS

Candida-Safe Recipes

1. Garlic and Herb Roasted Vegetables:

Ingredients:

Mixed vegetables (e.g., broccoli, cauliflower, bell peppers), olive oil, minced garlic, dried herbs (rosemary, thyme, oregano), salt, and pepper.

Instructions:

Toss vegetables with olive oil, garlic, herbs, salt, and pepper. Roast until tender.

2. Baked Lemon Herb Chicken:

Ingredients:

Chicken breasts or thighs, lemon juice, olive oil, fresh herbs (such as parsley and basil), minced garlic, salt, and pepper.

Instructions:

Marinate chicken in a mixture of lemon juice, olive oil, herbs, garlic, salt, and pepper. Bake until cooked through.

3. Quinoa and Vegetable Stir-Fry:

Ingredients:

Cooked quinoa, mixed vegetables, low-sodium soy sauce or tamari, minced garlic, ginger, and sesame oil.

Instructions:

Stir-fry vegetables with garlic, ginger, and a sauce made from soy sauce or tamari and sesame oil. Serve over cooked quinoa.

4. Zucchini Noodles with Pesto:

Ingredients:

Zucchini noodles (zoodles), homemade or store-bought pesto sauce (made with garlic, basil, olive oil, pine nuts, and nutritional yeast), cherry tomatoes.

Instructions:

Toss zucchini noodles with pesto sauce and halved cherry tomatoes for a fresh and satisfying dish.

5. Grilled Salmon with Avocado Salsa:

Ingredients:

Grilled salmon fillets, ripe avocados, diced tomatoes, red onion, cilantro, lime juice, salt, and pepper.

Instructions:

Make a salsa by combining diced avocados, tomatoes, red onion, cilantro, lime juice, salt, and pepper. Serve over grilled salmon.

6. Cucumber and Greek Yogurt Salad:

Ingredients:

Sliced cucumbers, Greek yogurt, minced garlic, fresh dill, lemon juice, salt, and pepper.

Instructions:

Toss sliced cucumbers with Greek yogurt, minced garlic, fresh dill, lemon juice, salt, and pepper for a refreshing salad.

7. Steamed Asparagus with Almond Butter Sauce:

Ingredients:

Fresh asparagus spears, almond butter, lemon juice, minced garlic, salt, and pepper.

Instructions:

Steam asparagus until tender. Prepare a sauce by mixing almond butter, lemon juice, garlic, salt, and pepper. Drizzle over asparagus.

8. Baked Sweet Potato Fries:

Ingredients:

Sweet potatoes, olive oil, paprika, garlic powder, salt, and pepper.

Instructions:

Cut sweet potatoes into fries, toss with olive oil and seasonings, and bake until crispy.

9. Spinach and Avocado Smoothie:

Ingredients:

Fresh spinach, ripe avocado, unsweetened almond milk, a squeeze of lemon juice, and a touch of stevia if desired.

Instructions:

Blend all ingredients until smooth for a nutrient-packed, low-sugar smoothie.

10. Broccoli and Leek Soup:

Ingredients:

Broccoli florets, leeks, garlic, vegetable broth, olive oil, salt, and pepper.

Instructions:

Sauté leeks and garlic in olive oil, add broccoli and vegetable broth, then simmer until the vegetables are tender. Blend until smooth for a creamy soup.

Meal Planning for Seniors

Day 1:

Breakfast:

- Oatmeal topped with sliced bananas and a sprinkle of chopped nuts
- A glass of low-fat milk or dairy-free alternative

Lunch:

- Grilled chicken salad with mixed greens, cherry tomatoes, cucumber, and a vinaigrette dressing
- Whole-grain roll or crackers.

Dinner:

- Baked salmon with lemon and dill
- Steamed broccoli and quinoa
- A small serving of mixed berries for dessert.

Day 2:

Breakfast:

- Greek yogurt with honey and fresh berries
- Whole-grain toast with a thin spread of almond butter

Lunch:

- Lentil soup with a side of mixed greens and a whole-grain roll

Dinner:

- Lean beef or vegetable stir-fry with brown rice
- Sautéed green beans with garlic.

Day 3:

Breakfast:

- Scrambled eggs with spinach and tomatoes
- A slice of whole-grain toast

Lunch:

- Tuna salad (or chickpea salad for a vegetarian option) in a whole-grain wrap
- A side of carrot sticks with hummus

Dinner:

- Roast the chicken with roasted sweet potatoes and Brussels sprouts.
- A small fruit salad for dessert.

Day 4:

Breakfast:

- Whole-grain waffles topped with low-fat yogurt and fresh peaches

Lunch:

- Vegetable and bean soup
- A whole-grain roll or crackers.

Dinner:

- Grilled shrimp or tofu with quinoa and vegetables
- Steamed asparagus.

Day 5:

Breakfast:

- Cottage cheese with sliced strawberries and a drizzle of honey
- A slice of whole-grain bread.

Lunch:

- Spinach and feta-stuffed chicken breast (or a vegetarian alternative)
- A side salad.

Dinner:

- Baked cod with a lemon and herb crust
- Steamed green beans and wild rice

Day 6:

Breakfast:

- Smoothie with spinach, banana, almond milk, and a scoop of protein powder

Lunch:

- Quinoa salad with mixed vegetables, chickpeas, and a tahini dressing

Dinner:

- Pork tenderloin with roasted butternut squash and sautéed kale

Day 7:

Breakfast:

- Scrambled eggs with diced bell peppers, onions, and a sprinkle of cheese
- Whole-grain toast.

Lunch:

- Minestrone soup with a side of mixed greens and a whole-grain roll

Dinner:

- Baked trout with a citrus glaze

- Quinoa pilaf and steamed broccoli

Day 9:

Breakfast:

- Whole-grain cereal with sliced strawberries and low-fat milk or a dairy-free alternative

Lunch:

- Turkey or tempeh sandwich on whole-grain bread with lettuce, tomato, and mustard
- A side of coleslaw

Dinner:

- Baked chicken thighs with a lemon and garlic marinade
- Roasted Brussels sprouts and quinoa

Day 10:

Breakfast:

- Cottage cheese and pineapple chunks
- A whole-grain muffin.

Lunch:

- Lentil and vegetable curry (or a vegetarian alternative) are served with brown rice.

Dinner:

- Grilled tilapia with mango salsa
- Steamed broccoli and couscous

Day 11:

Breakfast:

- Whole-grain pancakes with a dollop of Greek yogurt and fresh berries

Lunch:

- Spinach and mushroom omelet (or a tofu scramble for a vegetarian option)
- A side salad.

Dinner:

- Beef stew with a variety of vegetables
- A whole-grain dinner roll.

Day 12:

Breakfast:

- Smoothie with banana, kale, Greek yogurt, and a drizzle of honey

Lunch:

- Caprese salad with fresh tomatoes, mozzarella, basil, and balsamic glaze
- Whole-grain crackers.

Dinner:

- Baked cod with a tomato and olive tapenade
- Quinoa and steamed asparagus

Day 13:

Breakfast:

- Scrambled eggs with diced tomatoes, onions, and a sprinkle of grated cheese
- Whole-grain toast.

Lunch:

- Chickpea and vegetable stir-fry with a sesame ginger sauce
- Brown rice.

Dinner:

- Grilled pork loin with applesauce
- Roasted sweet potatoes and green beans

Day 14:

Breakfast:

- Whole-grain waffles topped with low-fat yogurt and mixed berries

Lunch:

- Tomato basil soup with a side of whole-grain bread

Dinner:

- Baked chicken or tofu with a honey mustard glaze
- Quinoa pilaf and sautéed kale

CHAPTER NINE

CANDIDA PREVENTION AND MAINTENANCE

Strategies for Preventing Recurrence

1. Follow a Candida-Friendly Diet: Continue to follow a diet that minimizes sugar, refined carbohydrates, and yeast-containing foods. Focus on whole, unprocessed foods, and emphasize lean proteins, vegetables, and complex carbohydrates.

2. Probiotics: Maintain a healthy gut microbiome by including probiotic-rich foods (e.g., yogurt with live cultures, kefir, sauerkraut) in your diet or by taking probiotic supplements. Probiotics can help keep Candida in check.

3. Limit Antibiotic Use: Use antibiotics only when necessary, and if prescribed, complete the full course. Antibiotics can disrupt the balance of gut bacteria, making it easier for Candida to overgrow.

4. Manage stress: Stress can weaken the immune system and contribute to Candida overgrowth. Incorporate stress-reduction techniques such as meditation, yoga, deep breathing, or hobbies that promote relaxation.

5. Maintain healthy blood sugar levels: Monitor and manage blood sugar levels if you have diabetes or prediabetes. Elevated blood sugar can promote Candida growth.

6. Stay Hydrated: Drink an adequate amount of water to support overall health and ensure proper digestion and detoxification.

7. Regular Exercise: Maintain a regular exercise routine to support immune function, improve circulation, and manage stress.

8. Limit Alcohol and Caffeine: Excessive alcohol and caffeine consumption can disrupt gut health. Consume these substances in moderation.

9. Oral Hygiene: Practice good oral hygiene, including regular brushing, flossing, and tongue cleaning. Candida can sometimes overgrow in the mouth, leading to oral thrush.

10. Get Adequate Sleep: Prioritize getting enough sleep, as sleep is crucial for immune function and overall health.

Long-Term Maintenance

1. Regular Check-Ups: Schedule regular check-ups with your healthcare provider to monitor your overall health and address any potential issues promptly.

2. Dietary Awareness: Maintain awareness of your dietary choices and their impact on your health. Be mindful of your sugar intake and continue to make choices that support gut health.

3. Listen to Your Body: Pay attention to any symptoms or changes in your health. If you notice recurring symptoms of Candida overgrowth, seek medical advice promptly.

4. Stay Informed: Stay informed about the latest research and developments related to Candida overgrowth and gut health. Knowledge can empower you to make informed choices.

5. Medication Management: If you're taking medications that may affect gut health, work closely with your healthcare provider to monitor their impact and explore alternatives if necessary.

6. Support Groups: Consider joining support groups or online communities focused on Candida's overgrowth. Connecting with others who have similar experiences can provide valuable insights and emotional support.

CONCLUSION

In conclusion, understanding Candida overgrowth and its potential impact on seniors' health is essential for effective prevention, management, and long-term well-being. Candida, a naturally occurring yeast, can become problematic when it overgrows, leading to a range of health issues. Seniors are particularly susceptible to Candida overgrowth due to age-related factors, weakened immune systems, and lifestyle factors.

Candida overgrowth can manifest with various symptoms, including digestive problems, fatigue, and recurrent infections. Recognizing these symptoms and understanding the role of Candida in the body is crucial for early intervention.

Seniors can take proactive steps to prevent and manage Candida overgrowth by adopting a Candida-friendly diet, incorporating antifungal herbs and supplements, practicing good nutritional support, and implementing stress reduction techniques and proper sleep hygiene.

Regular monitoring and assessment through medical tests and self-assessment tools can aid in identifying Candida overgrowth and its progression. Seek guidance from healthcare professionals for accurate diagnosis and treatment.

Long-term maintenance involves continued adherence to Candida-friendly dietary choices, stress management, and overall health practices. Regular check-ups, staying informed, and seeking professional advice when needed are key components of maintaining a healthy gut and overall well-being.

In the journey to prevent recurrence and maintain optimal health, individuals should focus on individualized care, dietary awareness, and listening to their bodies. By taking these measures, seniors can improve their quality of life, reduce the risk of Candida-related issues, and enjoy long-term health and vitality.

Printed in Great Britain
by Amazon